BACOPA MONNIERI FOR BEGINNERS

Unlocking Bacopa Monnieri, The Ultimate Guide To Cognitive Enhancement And Holistic Well-Being, Elevate Mental Clarity, Memory, And Health Naturally

Georgette Lockett

DISCLAIMER

The author of this book is not affiliated, associated, endorsed, sponsored, or approved by any company or individual. The views and opinions expressed in this book are solely those of the author and do not necessarily reflect the official policy or position of any entity.

The author hereby disclaims any relationship, collaboration, or partnership with any company or individual mentioned in this book. Any references to products, services, or individuals are provided for informational purposes only and should not be construed as an endorsement or recommendation.

Readers are advised to exercise their own judgment and discretion when applying the information provided in this book. The author shall not be held responsible for any actions taken by readers based on the content of this book.

This book is intended for general informational purposes only, and the author makes no representations or warranties of any kind, express or implied, about the completeness, accuracy, reliability, suitability, or availability of the information contained herein. Any reliance on the information in this book is at the reader's own risk.

The author reserves the right to update, change, or modify any information in this book without notice. It is the responsibility of the reader to verify any information before taking any actions based on the content of this book.

By reading this book, the reader acknowledges and agrees to the terms of this disclaimer.

Table of Contents

INTRODUCTION

Bacopa monnieri, often known as Brahmi or water hyssop, is a perennial plant endemic to wetlands around the globe, most notably in India, Australia, Europe, Africa, Asia, and North and South America. It's a beloved herb in Ayurveda, the old Indian medical system, for its profound therapeutic effects.

Brief Overview Of Bacopa Monnieri

Bacopa monnieri is distinguished by its tiny, succulent leaves and exquisite white or light purple blooms. It is often found growing in marshy places or near ponds and has been utilized in traditional medicine for ages due to its multiple health benefits. This plant's leaves contain active chemicals, particularly bacosides, which are thought to be responsible for its therapeutic properties. These bacosides have antioxidant effects that protect cells from free radical damage and may boost brain function.

Importance And Historical Use

This plant has a long history, most notably in Ayurveda, where it is regarded as a "Medhya Rasayana," or herb that improves memory and intelligence.

It has traditionally been used to improve cognitive performance, reduce anxiety, improve memory, and even cure epilepsy and asthma. Bacopa monnieri has been used in a variety of forms, including powders, teas, and extracts, and its effects have been recognized throughout generations, adding to its universal acceptance and usage.

Purpose And Structure

1. Chemical Composition and Active Chemicals: In this chapter, we will look at the individual chemicals present in Bacopa monnieri, concentrating on bacosides, alkaloids, flavonoids, and other elements that contribute to its therapeutic effects.

2. Health advantages: The emphasis of this section will be on the many health advantages linked with Bacopa monnieri, such as its influence on cognitive function, stress reduction, possible benefits for neurological illnesses, and role as an adaptogen.

3. Mode of Action and Mechanisms: This section will investigate how Bacopa monnieri interacts with the body, clarifying its mechanisms of action at the cellular and molecular levels to create therapeutic effects.

4. Clinical Studies and Research: This chapter will go over the current scientific literature and clinical studies that support the traditional applications of

Bacopa monnieri, as well as analyze the results, limits, and prospective future research areas.

5. Forms and Administration: The last chapter will discuss the various forms of Bacopa monnieri, suggested doses, and concerns for safe and effective administration.

These chapters will give a complete overview of Bacopa monnieri, from its historical origins and chemical makeup to its present usage and possible future implications in domains such as medicine, neurology, and wellness.

CHAPTER 1

Origins And Botanical Profile

Origin And Geographical Distribution

Bacopa monnieri, often known as Brahmi or Water Hyssop, is a perennial plant endemic to marshes and marshy places in India, Southeast Asia, and Australia. It is a member of the Plantaginaceae family and has a long history in traditional Ayurvedic treatment. The plant has evolved to survive in a broad range of conditions, from tropical to subtropical, and its spread is extensive.

Botanical Characteristics

Bacopa monnieri has succulent, creeping branches that grow horizontally and produce thick mats. The leaves are tiny, succulent, and oblong, arranged in an opposing pattern on the stem.

Depending on the cultivar, the plant produces tiny, five-petaled blooms that may be white, blue, or purple. The plant as a whole is recognized for its brilliant green color and thrives in watery situations, frequently partly immersed in water.

Growth Conditions And Cultivation

Bacopa monnieri is well-adapted to aquatic and semi-aquatic settings, making it a versatile plant that can grow in a variety of situations. It grows best in full to partial sunshine and in both stagnant and slow-flowing water. As long as the substrate is continually wet, the plant may survive in a variety of soil types, from sandy to clayey.

Seeds or cuttings may be used to cultivate Bacopa monnieri. Seeds are normally placed in a wet environment, and seedlings may be moved into appropriate sites once germinated. Cuttings are a typical technique of propagation, with stem segments forming roots when put in water or soil.

Watering regularly and nutrient-rich circumstances support healthy development.

Understanding Bacopa monnieri's botanical profile is critical for recognizing its adaptation and tenacity, which contribute to its global distribution and historical relevance. In the next chapters, we will look more into Bacopa monnieri, from its historical usage to its pharmacological qualities and present uses.

17

CHAPTER 2

Bioactive Compounds In Bacopa Monnieri

Identification Of Key Compounds

Brahmi, also known as Water Hyssop, has a large reservoir of bioactive chemicals that contribute to its medicinal qualities. Bacosides, alkaloids, flavonoids, saponins, and triterpenoid saponins are the major components responsible for their pharmacological actions. Bacosides A and B are the most recognized bioactive molecules, known for their neuroprotective and cognitive-enhancing properties.

Pharmacological Properties

1. Bacosides serve an important role in increasing neuronal function and guarding against neurodegeneration.

According to research, they have a role in boosting cognitive functioning, memory retention, and learning capacities by altering particular neurotransmitters, increasing nerve impulse transmission, and decreasing oxidative stress in the brain.

2. Antioxidant Activity: The bioactive components in Bacopa Monnieri have strong antioxidant activity, scavenging free radicals and decreasing oxidative stress. This antioxidant activity adds to its neuroprotective properties and may help to slow the aging process.

3. Research suggests that Bacopa Monnieri may have anxiolytic and anti-depressant effects via regulating neurotransmitters such as serotonin, dopamine, and GABA receptors, possibly reducing feelings of anxiety and sadness.

4. Anti-inflammatory characteristics: Certain chemicals in Bacopa Monnieri have anti-inflammatory characteristics, which may be effective in lowering inflammation in the body and perhaps boosting general health.

Impact On Health And Well-Being

The bioactive chemicals present in Bacopa Monnieri have the potential to provide a variety of health benefits, including:

• **Cognitive Enhancement:** Its ability to improve cognitive functioning, memory retention, and learning capacities makes it a promising treatment for brain health, particularly age-related cognitive decline.

• **Stress Reduction:** The adaptogenic qualities of Bacopa Monnieri may help with stress management and general mental well-being by possibly controlling stress hormone levels and supporting the body's stress response systems.

• **Neuroprotection:** The neuroprotective properties of Bacopa Monnieri's constituents make it a promising candidate for neurodegenerative illnesses and brain health protection.

• **Support for Overall Health:** Its antioxidant, anti-inflammatory, and perhaps anxiolytic characteristics add to its ability to promote overall health and vitality.

Understanding the bioactive components in Bacopa Monnieri and their pharmacological characteristics gives insight into its potential therapeutic uses in cognitive health, stress management, and general well-being. Further study is being conducted to investigate its mechanisms and possible uses in a variety of health fields.

CHAPTER 3

Traditional Uses And Cultural Significance

Bacopa Monnieri, a beloved plant in traditional medical systems such as Ayurveda, has a long history of diverse use throughout civilizations. Its traditional uses date back millennia and are deeply ingrained in the medical and cultural fabric of nations throughout the globe.

Historical Uses In Traditional Medicine

The Ancient Indian Healing System of Ayurveda:

Bacopa Monnieri, often known as Brahmi in Ayurveda, is revered for its cognitive-enhancing effects. It is classified as a "Medhya Rasayana," which is a plant that improves cognition, memory, and general brain function. Brahmi is used in formulas that promote mental clarity, focus, and nervous system support. It is said to help the mind balance, decrease stress, and boost cognitive capabilities.

Traditional Medical Practices Outside of India:

Bacopa Monnieri has been used in a variety of traditional medicinal practices outside of India. It is used in traditional Thai medicine for its adaptogenic characteristics, which are typically used to relieve stress and improve mental sharpness. Similarly, Bacopa has been utilized in traditional Chinese medicine to alleviate cognitive health concerns and increase general vigor.

Indigenous Methods:

Indigenous societies from Australia to South America have all recognized the therapeutic potential of Bacopa. It has been used to cure a variety of diseases in various forms—infusions, decoctions, or poultices—including respiratory disorders, skin conditions, and digestive issues.

Cultural Importance In Different Societies

Spiritual and medicinal value:

Bacopa Monnieri's therapeutic usefulness is recognized in many civilizations. It has spiritual value and is said to improve awareness and help meditation techniques. It is a valued plant among intellectuals, students, and spiritual searchers due to its relationship with mental clarity and heightened cognitive ability.

Integration in Everyday Life:

Bacopa's adaptability in treating mental well-being has led to its incorporation into daily living routines. Its use in traditional rituals, teas, and health regimens attests to its continued cultural significance.

Folklore And Anecdotes

Folk Traditions and Mythology:

Bacopa Monnieri is the subject of several cultural mythology and folklore. Brahmi is linked with the goddess Saraswati, the divinity of wisdom, music, and the arts, in Indian mythology. Consuming Brahmi is said to improve intellect and creative ability. Such legends have aided the herb's status as a sign of intelligence and innovation.

Legends and anecdotes:

Anecdotes and stories have been fashioned around Bacopa Monnieri throughout history, recounting its influence on cognitive capacities and lifespan. Brahmi's history includes stories of professors and sages employing the plant to strengthen their intellect and extend their mental sharpness.

Traditional applications and cultural importance of Bacopa Monnieri transcend geographical borders, indicating its long history of improving mental well-being and cognitive brilliance throughout many communities and historical eras.

CHAPTER 4

Scientific Research And Modern Applications

Contemporary Scientific Studies

In recent years, Bacopa Monnieri, often known as Brahmi, has been the focus of intense scientific investigation. The plant has a long history in traditional medicine, most notably in Ayurveda, and contemporary scientific investigations have attempted to elucidate its pharmacological effects. Researchers have concentrated on determining the active chemicals found in Bacopa Monnieri and how they affect different physiological systems.

One of the plant's purported cognitive-enhancing characteristics has piqued people's curiosity. Much research has been conducted to study the effects of Bacopa Monnieri on memory, learning, and cognitive function. Bacosides, the active chemicals, have been identified as the key contributors to these cognitive advantages. This research used a variety of approaches to investigate the influence of Bacopa Monnieri on memory retention, cognitive function, and neuroprotective effects, including animal models and human trials.

Furthermore, studies on the plant's antioxidant qualities have been conducted. Bacopa monnieri has been proven to have significant antioxidant activity, which is important for countering oxidative stress and protecting the brain from free radical damage. These results have ramifications for not just cognitive health, but also general well-being and lifespan.

Current Applications In Medicine And Health

The scientific insights gathered from Bacopa Monnieri's study have resulted in its incorporation into current medicine and health practices.

One well-known use is in neuropsychiatry. Bacopa Monnieri extracts and supplements are increasingly being utilized to maintain cognitive function and control aging-related diseases including memory loss and cognitive decline.

Furthermore, Bacopa Monnieri has made its way into formulations for stress and anxiety relief. According to research, the plant may contain anxiolytic properties that help people handle stress more successfully. This has mental health consequences and has spurred interest in Bacopa Monnieri as a natural alternative or supplemental treatment for anxiety disorders.

Bacopa Monnieri has long been utilized in traditional medical systems such as Ayurveda to treat a variety of illnesses such as epilepsy, asthma, and even some skin ailments. While current science is still investigating the veracity of some of these ancient claims, there is mounting evidence that the plant has adaptogenic and anti-inflammatory qualities.

Emerging Research Areas

Several promising study fields have attracted interest as the scientific community continues to investigate the possibilities of Bacopa Monnieri. One such field is research into its effect on neurodegenerative illnesses like Alzheimer's and Parkinson's. A preliminary study suggests that Bacopa Monnieri may have neuroprotective properties and more research is being conducted to determine the processes involved.

Another noteworthy element is the study of Bacopa Monnieri about mental disorders. Some studies have shown that it may have antidepressant properties, potentially via its effects on neurotransmitters and stress response pathways. More study is required to determine the effectiveness and safety of Bacopa Monnieri as a mood disorder treatment.

Finally, the path of Bacopa Monnieri from traditional medicine to modern science has been defined by increasing awareness of its various pharmacological characteristics. The plant's uses in cognitive health, stress management, and prospective functions in treating neurodegenerative illnesses and mood disorders keep it under investigation and offer promise for future therapeutic improvements.

CHAPTER 5

Mechanisms Of Action

How Bacopa Monnieri Works In The Body

Bacopa Monnieri's modes of action inside the body are complex and complicated. Bacosides, one of its key ingredients, have been extensively researched. These active chemicals have neuroprotective qualities, which help to protect neurons from injury and improve neurotransmitter transmission in the brain.

Bacopa monnieri interacts with many physiological systems, especially the central nervous system (CNS). It is thought to influence the actions of neurotransmitters such as acetylcholine, serotonin, and dopamine, all of which play important roles in cognition, mood control, and memory processing. Bacopa Monnieri may increase cognitive function, memory retention, and learning capacities by altering these neurotransmitter systems.

Interaction With Biological Systems

The interaction of the herb with biological systems extends beyond neurotransmitter regulation. Bacopa Monnieri contains antioxidants that scavenge free radicals and reduce oxidative stress. This function aids in the preservation of cellular integrity and the reduction of damage caused by oxidative stress, both of which may contribute to cognitive decline and a variety of neurodegenerative illnesses.

Furthermore, Bacopa Monnieri has been linked to neurogenesis or the production of new neurons in the brain. This impact adds to the herb's neuroprotective qualities and may improve cognitive health by assisting in brain cell repair and regeneration.

Effects On Cognitive Functions

Several studies have shown that Bacopa Monnieri may improve several elements of cognitive performance. Among the documented advantages include improved memory retention, learning capacity, and information processing speed. The herb's effect on neurotransmitters, in combination with its antioxidant and neuroprotective characteristics, adds to its beneficial effect on cognitive functioning.

Its effects on memory, especially long-term memory consolidation, have piqued the researchers' curiosity. Bacopa Monnieri has shown promise in memory development and retention, making it a potential treatment for age-related cognitive decline and illnesses such as Alzheimer's disease.

Understanding these methods of action sheds light on how Bacopa Monnieri exerts its cognitive-enhancing benefits, opening the door for future research into therapeutic uses as well as possible neuroprotective therapies.

As research into the processes and possible uses of Bacopa Monnieri continues, it provides intriguing pathways for the development of innovative treatments addressing cognitive health and neurological illnesses.

CHAPTER 6

Cognitive Enhancement And Neuroprotective Properties

Bacopa monnieri, also known as "Brahmi" in ancient Ayurvedic medicine, is a plant known for its cognitive-enhancing and neuroprotective characteristics. In Chapter 6, we look at the herb's diverse influence on cognitive function and its potential as a barrier against neurological degeneration.

Impact On Memory, Learning, And Cognition

Memory Improvement:

Bacopa Monnieri has been shown in studies to have a significant influence on memory enhancement. Its active components, notably bacosides, are attributed with increasing several elements of memory, including retention, recall, and information processing speed. Several studies have shown its effectiveness in improving both short-term and long-term memory capabilities. Notably, its benefits tend to build up over time, with longer periods of usage exhibiting more substantial cognitive gains.

Cognitive and Learning Function:

Beyond memory, Bacopa Monnieri has been shown to improve learning capacity and general cognitive function. It helps with attention span, concentration, and knowledge retention. According to research, consistent ingestion of Bacopa Monnieri may improve learning capacity, especially in difficult cognitive activities and information processing.

Neuroprotective Effects And Implications

Protecting Against Neurological Degeneration:

The neuroprotective capabilities of Bacopa Monnieri are one of its most fascinating features. It protects against aging-related cognitive decline and neurodegenerative disorders. According to research, its antioxidant capabilities aid in the fight against oxidative stress, lowering cellular damage and inflammation in the brain. By doing so, Bacopa Monnieri may reduce the risk of or halt the course of illnesses such as Alzheimer's and Parkinson's.

Neurological Health Implications:

The benefits of neuroprotection go beyond illness prevention. Bacopa Monnieri may benefit general brain health by promoting nerve cell development and maintenance. Its effect on neurotransmitters such as acetylcholine, serotonin, and dopamine promotes healthy brain function, influencing mood control, stress management, and mental clarity.

Clinical Trials And Findings

Clinical Research Evidence:

Clinical research on the cognitive benefits of Bacopa Monnieri has shown promising findings. These trials often lasted many weeks to months, demonstrating individuals' slow but constant increases in cognitive ability. These data support its use as a natural cognitive enhancer and neuroprotectant.

Real-World Examples:

Because of the implications of Bacopa Monnieri's cognitive advantages, it has been used in a variety of supplements and nootropic compositions. The fact that it is widely available as a supplement demonstrates its perceived efficacy in boosting cognitive well-being and brain health.

In conclusion, Chapter 6 sheds light on Bacopa Monnieri's critical role in increasing cognitive capabilities, bolstering the brain's defensive systems, and perhaps providing a barrier against neurological degeneration. Its diverse activities make it an attractive topic for future investigation, opening the path for novel methods for cognitive improvement and neurological wellness.

CHAPTER 7

Mood Regulation And Stress Alleviation

Bacopa Monnieri, a respected plant in traditional medicine, has effects that go beyond cognitive improvement and into mood management and stress relief. This chapter dives into the many facets of Bacopa Monnieri's emotional well-being, stress management, and underlying psychological processes.

Influence On Mood And Emotional Well-Being

The possible influence of Bacopa Monnieri on mood and emotional states is one of its most fascinating elements. Traditional medical systems, notably Ayurveda, have long acknowledged its capacity to improve emotional balance and general well-being.

Scientific studies have attempted to elucidate the neurochemical basis of these effects.

According to research, Bacopa Monnieri may affect neurotransmitters including serotonin, dopamine, and gamma-aminobutyric acid (GABA), all of which play important roles in mood regulation. Bacopa Monnieri may lead to a more stable and good emotional state by affecting these neurotransmitter systems. The adaptogenic qualities of the herb, which help the body adapt to stimuli, are thought to contribute to its mood-regulating benefits.

Stress-Relieving Properties

The historical usage of Bacopa Monnieri as an adaptogen gives a good framework for understanding its stress-relieving qualities. In today's world, when chronic stress is a major problem, the herb's ability to reduce the physiological and psychological effects of stress is of significant importance.

According to research, Bacopa Monnieri may influence the levels of stress hormones like cortisol in the body. Cortisol, sometimes known as the "stress hormone," is essential in the body's reaction to stress. Bacopa Monnieri may help minimize the detrimental effects of chronic stress on several physiological systems, including the cardiovascular and immunological systems, by controlling cortisol levels.

Psychological Effects And Mechanisms

Bacopa Monnieri's psychological benefits go beyond cognitive improvement to include mood and stress modulation. The interaction of the herb with neurotransmitter systems, neurotrophic factors, and antioxidant pathways helps to explain its psychological advantages.

The ability of Bacopa Monnieri to improve brain connectivity and induce neuroplasticity may be related to its mood-regulating properties. The capacity of the brain to remodel itself and generate new synaptic connections, known as neuroplasticity, is critical for adaptive responses to stress and emotional events.

Furthermore, Bacopa Monnieri's antioxidant qualities may protect the brain from oxidative stress, which has been linked to mood disorders and neurodegenerative illnesses. The herb may help the general resilience of the brain against diverse stresses by lowering oxidative damage.

The seventh chapter delves into the complex link between Bacopa Monnieri and psychological well-being. The plant comprehensively promotes mental health, from mood management to stress reduction. The processes behind these psychological impacts are anticipated to be further explained as scientific research proceeds, opening the path for improved applications in mental health and well-being.

CHAPTER 8

Dosage, Safety, And Side Effects

Recommended Dosage Guidelines

The recommended dose of Bacopa Monnieri depends on several variables, including the intended usage, individual tolerance, and the supplement's exact formulation. Standardized extracts often recommend doses ranging from 300mg to 450mg daily, with at least 55% bacosides—the main components in Bacopa linked with its cognitive benefits.

The effectiveness of Bacopa Monnieri, on the other hand, seems to increase gradually over many weeks of constant administration. As a result, some suggestions advocate for a greater first dose, followed by a maintenance dose. To establish the optimum dose for individual requirements, it is critical to follow manufacturer directions or speak with a healthcare expert.

Safety Considerations

Bacopa Monnieri has a positive safety record when taken at approved dosages. Certain safeguards, however, are urged. Because of the possibility of interactions, pregnant or nursing women, as well as those with certain medical problems or taking drugs, should see a healthcare practitioner before using Bacopa supplements.

Potential Side Effects And Precautions

While most people handle Bacopa Monnieri well, some people may develop moderate side effects such as nausea, upset stomach, dry mouth, or exhaustion. These effects are usually temporary and fade with prolonged usage. Some people may have allergic responses on rare occasions.

Long-term safety evidence is inadequate, therefore use with care over time, particularly at larger dosages. It is important to keep an eye out for any negative effects and to be aware of individual sensitivities.

To assure quality and purity, get Bacopa Monnieri pills from trustworthy vendors. Furthermore, following suggested doses and communicating any concerns with a healthcare expert will help reduce possible dangers.

Understanding Bacopa Monnieri's dose, safety concerns, and potential side effects is critical for maximizing its advantages while reducing any potential hazards. Before beginning supplements, always emphasize educated decision-making and contact with a healthcare practitioner, particularly if you have underlying health concerns or are using drugs.

CHAPTER 9

Comparative Analysis And Formulations

Comparison With Other Cognitive Supplements

Because of its long history of usage and scientific support, Bacopa Monnieri stands out among cognitive supplements. Its unique mode of action distinguishes it from other supplements, as it improves cognitive processes via many routes, including memory improvement and neuroprotection.

When compared to common cognitive supplements such as Ginkgo Biloba and Ginseng, Bacopa Monnieri has different effects. While Ginkgo Biloba is known for its blood circulation and antioxidant properties, Bacopa Monnieri's main functions include improving synaptic transmission, increasing neurotransmitter balance, and countering the effects of stress on cognitive performance. Each supplement has unique characteristics and focused effects on cognitive health.

Different Formulations And Variations

Supplements containing Bacopa Monnieri are available in a variety of forms, including capsules, powders, extracts, and tinctures. The concentration and bioavailability of these formulations may vary. For consistency and effectiveness, standardized extracts containing particular percentages of active chemicals, such as bacosides, are often recommended.

The concentration of bacosides, the active ingredients in Bacopa Monnieri, differs across formulations. Increased potency is often associated with higher bacoside concentration. The extraction procedure also has an impact on the final product's composition and efficacy. Some formulations incorporate additional substances to boost bioavailability or supplement the benefits of Bacopa Monnieri.

Synergistic Effects With Other Compounds

According to research, when taken with specific chemicals, Bacopa Monnieri may have synergistic benefits. For example, combining it with other adaptogenic herbs such as Ashwagandha or Rhodiola Rosea may increase its stress-relieving qualities and general cognitive advantages. Furthermore, combining Bacopa Monnieri with nutrients such as Omega-3 fatty acids or antioxidants may enhance its neuroprotective benefits.

Understanding the interactions and synergies of Bacopa Monnieri with other chemicals enables the development of more effective formulations or supplementation regimens customized to particular cognitive or health demands.

Finally, the unique processes, different formulations, and possible interactions with other compounds of Bacopa Monnieri allow a wide spectrum for investigating its uses and improving its cognitive and health advantages. Continuous research and comparative analysis may assist in enhancing its use and uncover new avenues for improving cognitive functioning and general well-being.

CHAPTER 10

Future Prospects And Conclusion

Future Directions In Research

With its extensive historical usage and potential modern study discoveries, Bacopa Monnieri remains a topic of interest for scientists and researchers. Future research will most likely go further into various elements of Bacopa Monnieri, investigating new dimensions and broadening our knowledge. Some probable future study directions include:

1. While the mechanisms of action of Bacopa Monnieri have been researched, there is still potential for a more in-depth study of its interactions with different biological systems. Uncovering the specific molecular mechanisms involved in its effects on cognition and

neuroprotection may open the way for tailored treatment therapies.

2. Long-Term Effects: Long-term usage of Bacopa Monnieri is critical for evaluating its safety and effectiveness over time. Long-term research might shed light on its long-term cognitive advantages and possible changes inside the body.

3. Diversity in Clinical Studies: Extending clinical studies to include various people might give insight into any differences in Bacopa Monnieri's effects depending on age, gender, or underlying health issues. This inclusion would lead to a better understanding of its application across various groups.

4. Combination Studies: Researching the synergistic benefits of Bacopa Monnieri when combined with other cognitive-enhancing substances might be a fascinating field of study. Understanding how it interacts with other adaptogens and nootropics may open up new avenues for cognitive improvement.

Potential Advancements And Innovations

As research advances, various developments and innovations linked to Bacopa Monnieri are possible:

1. **Enhancement of Bioavailability:** Creating formulations that increase the bioavailability of Bacopa Monnieri's active components might improve its overall efficacy. This might include new delivery mechanisms or co-administration with substances that improve absorption.

2. **Customized Formulations:** Tailoring formulations to individual demands and health profiles might become a trend. Combining Bacopa Monnieri with additional herbs or minerals might result in tailored cognitive improvement regimens.

3. **Integration with Technology:** As digital health becomes more prevalent, there may be novel techniques for incorporating Bacopa Monnieri into digital health platforms, integrating traditional

herbal therapies with contemporary technology for individualized health management.

Summary Of Key Findings And Conclusions

Finally, Bacopa Monnieri is a versatile plant with a rich past and a bright future. This in-depth examination of its origins, botanical profile, mechanisms of action, and many uses emphasizes its importance in cognitive improvement and neuroprotection.

The scientific literature evaluated in this research indicates the beneficial effects of Bacopa Monnieri on cognitive processes, mood control, and stress relief. Its possible neuroprotective capabilities provide a further layer of significance, with larger implications for brain health.

However, it is critical to approach the usage of Bacopa Monnieri with knowledge of its suggested doses, safety concerns, and potential adverse effects.

Future studies in these areas should continue to deepen our understanding, guaranteeing the appropriate and successful use of Bacopa Monnieri in health and wellness practices.

The dynamic landscape of cognitive enhancement research is expected to see exciting advances in the future, with Bacopa Monnieri playing a vital part in determining the future of brain health and well-being.

Conclusion

It is important to reflect on the entire information obtained through the various chapters before ending the investigation of Bacopa Monnieri. This extraordinary plant has withstood the test of time and continues to reveal its numerous advantages in recent scientific investigations.

Recap Of Essential Points Discussed

1. **Origins and Botanical Profile:** Bacopa Monnieri, which is endemic to wetlands around the globe, has special botanical characteristics and flourishes under certain growing circumstances. Its flexibility and durability help to explain why it is so widely grown.

2. Extensive scientific study has been conducted throughout the years into the many uses of Bacopa Monnieri in medicine and health. Its medicinal potential has been supported by empirical data ranging from memory improvement to stress reduction.

3. **Mechanisms of Action:** Discovering how Bacopa Monnieri interacts with biological systems has shown its complex influence on cognitive functioning. Its regulation of neurotransmitters and

antioxidative capabilities contribute greatly to its cognitive-enhancing benefits.

4. Cognitive Enhancement and Neuroprotective Properties: Clinical investigations have proven Bacopa Monnieri's remarkable influence on memory, learning, and cognition, as well as its neuroprotective properties, pointing to its promise in enhancing brain health and cognitive lifespan.

5. Mood Regulation and Stress Reduction: The herb's capacity to favorably regulate mood and reduce stress has aroused interest in its psychological effects, giving light to its potential as an adaptogen and mood stabilizer.

6. Dosage, Safety, and Side Effects: Understanding the recommended dosage, safety concerns, and possible side effects is critical for reaping the advantages of Bacopa Monnieri while remaining safe.

7. Comparative Analysis and Formulations: Comparing Bacopa Monnieri to other cognitive supplements, experimenting with different formulations, and researching its synergistic effects with other chemicals all contribute to a better understanding of its distinctiveness and potential in many situations.

8. Future Prospects and Conclusion: The future of Bacopa Monnieri's research is bright. Continuing research might lead to the discovery of novel applications, formulations, and deeper mechanistic insights, opening the path for new uses and advances.

Conclusions on the Importance and Potential of Bacopa Monnieri

The path of Bacopa Monnieri from Ayurvedic traditions to current scientific investigation has shown its enormous promise as a cognitive enhancer, stress reducer, and neuroprotective agent.

Its importance stems not just from its established advantages, but also from the continual research of its undiscovered potential.

The versatility of this herb, together with its numerous therapeutic benefits on the brain and emotional well-being, makes it a potential natural supplement. The capacity of Bacopa Monnieri to favorably affect cognition, mood, and stress response provides a comprehensive approach to mental well-being.

As research into the complicated processes and uses of Bacopa Monnieri continues, it remains a beacon of hope for people looking for natural therapies to improve cognitive functioning and increase mental well-being. The combination of traditional knowledge and current scientific confirmation highlights Bacopa Monnieri's lasting potential in determining the future of brain health and cognitive development. Embracing this botanical jewel while keeping dose and safety standards in mind may pave the path for a better, healthier future enhanced by nature's offerings.

THE END